FRED SWISMAN

Type 1 Diabetes

A Guide for Parents

First edition

This book was professionally typeset on Reedsy.
Find out more at reedsy.com

To our little heroes,their families & caregivers.

In honor of World Diabetes Day.

Contents

Preface

Dear Parents,

When you have children with type 1 diabetes (T1D), you are instantly faced with the often difficult responsibility of parenting a child while assisting them in navigating life with a chronic condition. Guilt, worry, and dread are only the peak of the iceberg. There will be nights spent awake testing your child's blood sugar to ensure that they are not hypoglycemic (low blood sugar), and days spent thinking about lunchtime at your child's school.

I realize how frightening it may be, and I created this book in the hopes of shedding more light on this illness. And to show you that you are not alone in this.

1

Learning About Diabetes

Diabetes is a disorder in which the body's capacity to process blood glucose, often known as blood sugar, is impaired. Diabetes is classified into different categories, each with its own set of treatment. It is a chronic condition that happens when the pancreas does not create enough insulin or when the body cannot adequately utilize the insulin that is produced. Insulin is a hormone that controls blood glucose levels. Hyperglycemia, also known as high blood glucose or elevated blood sugar, is a typical side effect of untreated diabetes that, over time, causes substantial damage to a number of the body's systems, particularly the neurons and blood vessels.

In the United States, an estimated 34.2 million people of all ages have diabetes, both diagnosed and undiagnosed.

Digestion is the method by which you breakdown the food you ingest into numerous nutritional sources. When you eat carbs (such as bread, rice, or pasta), your body converts them into sugar (glucose). When glucose enters your bloodstream, it requires assistance - a "key" - to reach its eventual destination, that is inside your body's cells (cells comprise of your body's tissues and organs). Insulin is this "help" or "key." Insulin is a hormone made by your pancreas, an organ located behind your stomach. Your pancreas releases insulin into your bloodstream. Insulin acts as the "key" that unlocks the cell wall "door," which allows glucose to enter your body's cells. Glucose provides the "fuel" or energy tissues and organs need to properly function. Not being able to produce insulin leads to diabetes.

Types of Diabetes

According to the World Health Organization "Diabetes caused a 3% rise in age-standardized death rates between 2000 and 2019. Diabetes-related mortality increased by 13% in lower-middle-income nations ". Diabetes can be classified into the following types:

Gestational Diabetes *:* Some women develop this kind throughout their pregnancy. Gestational diabetes normally disappears after the pregnancy. However, if you have gestational diabetes, you are more likely to acquire Type 2 diabetes later in life.

Type 2 Diabetes: This kind occurs when your body either does not produce enough insulin or when your cells do not respond appropriately to insulin. This is the most prevalent kind of diabetes. Type 2 diabetes affects up to 95% of diabetics. It commonly affects persons in their forties and fifties. Type 2 diabetes is also known as adult-onset diabetes and insulin-resistant diabetes. "Having a bit of sugar" is what your parents or grandparents could have described it as.

Prediabetes: This is the phase before Type 2 diabetes. The blood sugar levels are above normal, but not high enough to be diagnosed as having Type 2 diabetes.

In the following chapter, we will go into type 1 diabetes in children in further detail.

2

Type 1 Diabetes

According to the American Diabetes Association, 1.6 million individuals with type 1 diabetes, including about 187,000 children and adolescents.

Type 1 diabetes (formerly known as insulin-dependent, juvenile, or childhood-onset diabetes) is characterized by insufficient insulin production and need daily insulin administration. In most patients with type 1 diabetes, the body's immune system, which ordinarily fights infection, assaults and kills insulin-producing cells in the pancreas. As a result,the pancreas ceases to produce insulin. Glucose cannot enter the cells without insulin, causing blood glucose to increase above normal. Persons may use injections or an insulin pump to do this. There were 9 million persons with type 1 diabetes in 2017, with the majority of them living in high-income nations. Its cause and prevention methods are unknown as of now. A person with type 1 diabetes may be diagnosed while they are young. To control type 1 diabetes, patients must periodically monitor their blood sugar levels, take insulin, and make some lifestyle adjustments. Although both types of diabetes (type 1 & 2) can arise in children, this illness is distinct from type 2 diabetes. Both kinds have symptoms that are comparable.

Who is at a higher risk of developing type 1 diabetes?

Type 1 diabetes is most common in children and young adults, but it can appear at any age. Having a diabetic parent or sibling increases your chances of having type 1 diabetes. Type 1 diabetes affects around 5% of diabetics in the United States.

What Causes Type 1 Diabetes in Some People?

Nobody knows for certain why certain people have type 1 diabetes. Doctors and scientists believe it is caused by a person's genes. However, simply possessing the diabetes genes is unlikely to be sufficient. Something else is most likely required. Scientists are investigating if additional factors, such as certain viral infections, a person's birth weight, or their nutrition, may cause someone who already possesses the genes for type 1 diabetes more likely to develop it.

What Factors Influence Blood Sugar Levels?

Blood sugar levels can be affected by a variety of factors. Some are difficult to regulate, such as disease, stress, and hormones. Food, medicine, and exercise are examples of things you and your child can learn to control. The care staff will discuss these with you frequently.

·Food: Carbohydrates in diet elevate blood sugar naturally. As a result, the types and quantity of foods your child consumes might have an impact. To assist you, your care team will make meal and snack suggestions.

·Insulin: Diabetes medications, such as insulin, which decreases blood sugar levels, also have an effect on blood sugar levels. You'll figure out how to balance it with the meals your youngster consumes. Your medical team will educate you how to use insulin and when to change it.

·Exercise: Keeping active is beneficial for children with type 1 diabetes. Exercise decreases blood sugar levels and keeps children fit. Determine the best strategy for your child to be active while keeping their blood sugar levels as stable as possible.

Fact: *Hypoglycemia occurs when a person's blood sugar becomes too low. This requires immediate attention. Hyperglycemia is an elevated blood sugar level. Untreated hyperglycemia can progress to diabetic ketoacidosis, which likewise need immediate medical attention. Inquire with your medical team about these problems and what to look out for.*

What Happens If Blood Sugar Levels Are Too High or Too Low?

Even if you follow the care plan and closely monitor your child's blood sugar, he or she may experience high or low blood sugars on occasion. Blood sugar levels might be affected by eating too much on a particular occasion or exercising more or less than usual.

Hypoglycemia occurs when a person's blood sugar becomes too low. This requires immediate attention. Hyperglycemia is a high blood sugar level. Untreated hyperglycemia can progress to diabetic ketoacidosis, which likewise need immediate medical attention. Inquire with your medical team about these problems and what to look out for. Maintaining good blood sugar levels benefits your child both now and in the future. Maintaining stable and balanced blood sugar levels today may reduce your child's risk of developing health problems during adolescence and into adulthood.

Make use of your care team for assistance. They will assist you in improving your knowledge and confidence in managing your child's diabetes.

Symptoms of Type 1 Diabetes

Most people's symptoms of type 1 diabetes are similar, although teens and adults are more likely to recognize them. Type 1 diabetes can develop gradually or suddenly. Sometimes children might not develop diabetic symptoms until blood or urine tests are performed for another cause. Children who exhibit symptoms may:

- start wetting the bed after sleeping dry
- increased thirst and urine
- impaired eyesight
- exhaustion
- unexplained weight loss
- increased appetite

These symptoms usually appear quickly across a few days to weeks. Frequent urination and thirst are frequent early symptoms of diabetes in children. They may also appear more annoyed and agitated than normal.

Diabetic ketoacidosis can cause the start of type 1 diabetes symptoms (DKA). This is a significant issue in which the body enters a condition of ketosis due to a shortage of glucose entering the cells. This is when the body begins to break down fats into acids known as ketones for energy.

DKA is considered a medical emergency. Symptoms could include:

- vomiting or nausea
- skin that is dry or flushed
- sweet-smelling breath
- breathing difficulties
- stomach ache
- thinking difficulties

Causes

Type 1 diabetes is an autoimmune condition in which the immune system targets healthy cells in the body. These are the insulin-producing beta cells found in the pancreas in type 1 diabetes.

It is unknown what causes the immune system to target pancreatic cells. Some genetic factors can raise the likelihood of developing type 1 diabetes. People who have either HLA-DR3-DQ2 or HLA-DR4-DQ8 genes, or both, are more likely to develop type 1 diabetes. If a parent has type 1 diabetes, a child's chance of acquiring the disease ranges from 1 in 17 to 1 in 25.

Diagnosis

Anyone who has a child who is showing signs or symptoms of diabetes should take them to the doctor for a checkup. If you notice any of the symptoms of DKA, you should call 911 right away. Children with type 1 diabetes are frequently seen by a **pediatric endocrinologist**. This type of specialist detects and treats hormone-related issues such as diabetes.

A blood test will be required to diagnose type 1 diabetes. These tests can assess a variety of body systems that may suggest diabetes. To diagnose type 1 diabetes, most doctors will utilize a random plasma glucose test. This entails assessing blood sugar levels at the time of testing. Diabetes is diagnosed when blood sugar levels exceed 200 milligrams per deciliter (mg/dl).

Other tests can be used by healthcare practitioners to detect diabetes. Fasting blood sugar tests, which require no food the night before, are one example. The

A1C test measures the average blood sugar levels over the previous few months. Glucose tolerance tests assess blood sugar levels before and after consuming a glucose-containing beverage. If a doctor suspects type 1 diabetes, they may additionally test for auto antibodies. These are chemicals that indicate the immune system is targeting healthy tissues in the body. A urine sample may also be tested for ketones. Auto antibodies are not present in the blood of people with type 2 diabetes, and ketones in the urine are improbable.

How Is Blood Sugar Determined?

The blood sugar levels of your child will inform you how effectively the care plan is functioning. Blood sugar may be measured in two ways:

Daily blood sugar levels: These are the readings you take throughout the day with a glucose meter. If your kid is wearing a continuous glucose monitor, the blood sugar level can be seen on the display at any time.

Blood sugar levels in recent months:

You'll meet with the care team every few months, and they'll send your child for a blood test named glycosylated hemoglobin (hemoglobin A1c or HbA1c). The findings will reveal how frequently your child's blood glucose levels were in and out of the normal range in the 2-3 months before the test.

At your child's frequent diabetes checks, you'll review blood sugar readings with the care team, and they'll change the treatment plan as appropriate.

4

Treatment & Complications

Because there is no cure for type 1 diabetes yet, it must be treated for the rest of one's life. A diabetic care plan is used by doctors to treat type 1 diabetes. The care plan instructs you and your kid on how to maintain appropriate blood sugar levels on a daily basis.

Each child's diabetic treatment plan is tailored to their specific needs. However, all plans contain the same four essential components:

- use insulin (by injection or an insulin pump)
- consume a healthy, balanced diet that involves carb counting
- Check your child's blood sugar levels at least four times each day.
- participate in frequent physical activity

To control their blood sugar levels, children with type 1 diabetes will require daily insulin injections. This might be accomplished using a syringe, pump, or insulin pen. Insulin is not available in tablet form because stomach acid would degrade it too rapidly.

Some youngsters will be unable to achieve a healthy blood sugar level only with the use of insulin. In certain circumstances, doctors may prescribe diabetic medicines, such as pramlintide, to be taken in conjunction with insulin. Doctors will also advise you to monitor your blood sugar levels on a frequent basis to avoid issues.

Complications

Over time, type 1 diabetes can lead to major health issues, including :
    Cardiovascular Disease
    Stroke
    Kidney Disorder
    Dentistry And Vision Issues
    Injury To The Nerves
    Foot Issues
    Depression
    Obstructive Sleep Apnea
The most common cause of type 1 diabetes symptoms is DKA, which is a medical emergency. Parents and other caregivers who notice any of the symptoms of DKA should take the child right away to the hospital for treatment.

5

Caring For a TD1 Child

If your child or adolescent has type 1 diabetes, the next step is to commence treatment. Diabetes treatment include maintaining appropriate blood sugar levels. Your child's diabetes care team will treat them according to a specific diabetes care plan created just for them.

Diabetes is being researched and treated by researchers and clinicians all around the world. Up until then, maintaining a treatment schedule is essential to managing diabetes and living a long, healthy life.

Taking Blood Sugar Readings

Blood sugar levels must be monitored daily as part of type 1 diabetes treatment. There are two approaches to this:

~Using a glucose meter: Most children with type 1 diabetes must monitor their blood sugar levels before meals and before going to bed. This happens four times a day, sometimes more. The care plan will inform you how often to check your child's blood sugar and what to do if it is too high or too low.

~With the aid of a continuous glucose monitor (CGM): This wearable gadget checks blood sugar levels every few minutes during the day and night. It employs a thread-like sensor that is inserted beneath the skin and fixed in place. Sensors can be left in place for up to 10 days before needing to be changed. Because a CGM measures blood sugar so frequently, it can assist you and your care team in doing an even better job of keeping sugar levels in the healthy range.

The blood sugar readings will be used by the care team to adapt your child's insulin regimen over time.

Using Insulin

All children and adolescents with type 1 diabetes must take insulin in order for glucose to enter their cells and provide energy. Your child's insulin regimen will be customized by the care team.

~Insulin can be administered to children by injection: Every day, children often require four or more shots. An insulin needle is quite little, and an injection is not uncomfortable. Your child's care team will educate you how to assist him or her deal with injections.

~Using an insulin pump: The pump constantly injects insulin into the body through a tiny tube implanted just beneath the skin.

Healthy Eating

To keep their blood sugars in a safe range, children with type 1 diabetes must find the correct combination of diet, insulin, and activity. It is beneficial to understand how different meals impact your child's blood sugar levels. The care staff will educate you how to eat properly and how to count carbohydrates in meals and snacks. When you know how many carbohydrates your child consumes, you can calculate how much insulin they require. This allows your child the freedom to eat whenever and as much they want.

Engaging in Regular Physical Activity

Exercise builds your child's muscles and bones, improves their mood, and regulates their blood sugar levels. In fact, being active improves insulin function. Type 1 diabetic children can and should exercise.

Managing Your Child's Sugar Levels

Getting blood sugars into a healthy range might be difficult at first. However, you and your child will eventually take responsibility of diabetes together. Here are some pointers:

1. Learn everything you can about diabetes and your child's treatment plan. You can ask the care team any question you want. They are glad to assist you and answer any queries.
2. Blood tests and medications should be administered to your child. Check your child's blood sugar levels on a regular basis. Assure that your child takes insulin or other diabetic medications as directed.
3. Stick to the food plan:Provide meals and snacks that complement your child's meal plan, with an emphasis on providing a variety of healthful options.
4. Encourage mobility and exercise: Encourage your youngster to participate in physical activity on a regular basis.
5. Get regular physicals:Ensure that your child has frequent checks with the care staff.

Developing good habits and routines with your kid will aid in the management of their diabetes. Your efforts will help keep your children healthy.

6

Monitoring Sugar Levels

Why Should Blood Sugars Be Checked?

Checking your child's blood sugar shows you how much glucose (glucose level) is in his or her blood and is an important aspect of everyday care. Every time you check, you'll know if your child's blood sugar is inside or beyond the healthy range specified by the care team.

- Regular blood sugar checks can assist you and your child:
- Have better control of diabetes.
- Learn how diet, exercise, and diabetes medication impact blood sugar levels.
- Know when to make adjustments to your diet, exercise, and diabetes medications.
- Take care of sick days.
- Prevent health problems from occurring now or in the future.

When Should I Have My Child's Blood Sugar Checked?

When to monitor your child's blood sugar will be determined by the diabetes care team. Most children and adolescents should be tested before each meal, before going to bed, and before, during, and after activities.

Even if your child is asleep, there are situations when you may need to test more frequently. For instance, suppose your child has recently been diagnosed with diabetes.

- Your youngster is unwell.
- Your child's blood sugar levels are frequently high or low.
- Your child's diabetic treatment or everyday routines have changed.

What Instrument Do I Use to Check Blood Sugar?

As previously stated, there are two types of instruments that can measure blood sugar or glucose levels:

A blood glucose meter detects the quantity of glucose in the blood, whereas a continuous glucose monitor detects the amount of glucose in the fluid surrounding the cells immediately beneath the skin.

Your kid's care team can advise you on the ideal gadget for your child.

What Happens When the Tests Are Completed?

When necessary, your child's health care team can access the data online or during clinic appointments. They will examine your child's glucose levels for trends, such as high or low sugars at specific times of the day. Patterns can assist doctors in adjusting medications and dietitians in making dietary modifications.

Try not to get disappointed if your child's glucose level is higher or lower than you expect from time to time. Inquire with your child's care team about any modifications you should make. You'll discover out how to keep your child's sugar levels as close to normal as possible.

7

End Note

The thorough care plan and diabetes care team helps keep you on track as you assist your child in managing type 1 diabetes. The best method to keep your kids healthy is to stick to the plan and communicate regularly with the care team. Join support groups to learn more about the illness and to have a group of people who understand your challenges as a parent caring for a kid with TD1.

Also by Fred Swisman

Pneumonia is one of the ninth leading cause of mortality in the United States particularly in children. Learn more about this disease it's symptoms, diagnosis & treatment.

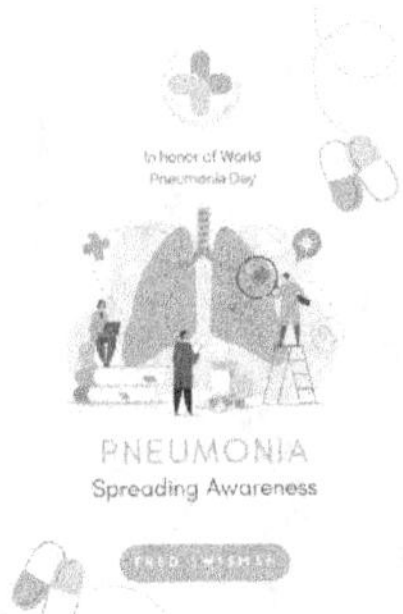

Pneumonia : Spreading Awareness

Available on Amazon.